PLANT BASED DIET COOKBOOK 2021 FOR BEGINNERS

50 easy, fast and mouth-watering recipes for everyday meals. Lose up to 5 pounds in 5 days with simple steps.

Ursa Males

TABLE OF CONTENTS

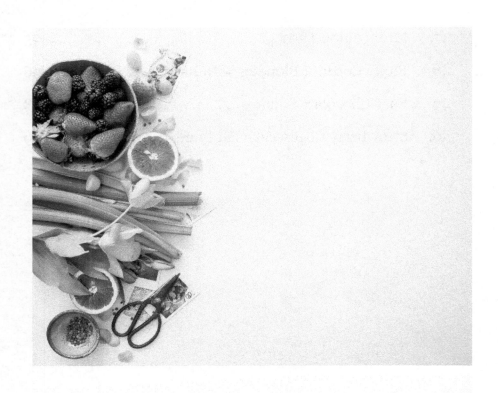

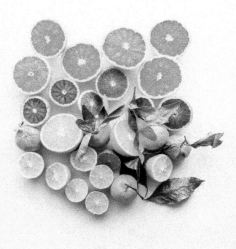

BREAKFAST

1. **Simple Garlic and Kale**

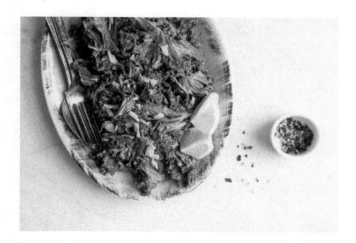

Preparation time: 5 minutes

Cooking time: 10 minutes

Servings: 4

Ingredients:

- 1 bunch kale
- 2 tablespoons olive oil
- 4 garlic cloves, minced

Directions:

1. Carefully tear the kale into bite-sized portions, making sure to remove the stem. Discard the stems. Take a large-sized pot and place it over medium heat

2. Add olive oil and let the oil heat up. Add garlic and stir for 2 minutes. Add kale and cook for 5-10 minutes. Serve!

Nutrition: Calories: 121 Fat: 8g Carbohydrates: 5g Protein: 4g

2. Crispy Morning Tofu

Preparation time: 5 minutes

Cooking time: 30 minutes

Servings: 8

Ingredients:

- 1-pound extra-firm tofu, drained and sliced
- 2 tablespoons olive oil
- 1 cup almond meal
- 1 tablespoon yeast
- ½ teaspoon onion powder
- ½ teaspoon garlic powder
- ½ teaspoon oregano
- ¼ teaspoon salt

Directions:

1. Add all ingredients except the tofu and olive oil in a shallow bowl. Mix well. Preheat your oven to 400 degrees Fahrenheit.
2. In a wide bowl, add the almond meal and mix well. Brush tofu with olive oil, dip into the mix, and coat well. Line a baking sheet with parchment paper.

3. Transfer coated tofu to the baking sheet. Bake within 20-30 minutes, making sure to flip once until golden brown. Serve and enjoy!

Nutrition: Calories: 282 Fat: 20g Carbohydrates: 9g Protein: 12g

3. Chia Coffee Mix

Preparation time: 15 minutes

Cooking time: 0 minutes

Servings: 1

Ingredients:

- 1 tablespoon chia seeds
- 2 cups strongly brewed coffee, chilled
- 1 ounce Macadamia nuts
- 1-2 packets Stevia, optional
- 1 tablespoon MCT oil

Directions:

1. Add all the listed ingredients to a blender. Blend on high until smooth and creamy. Enjoy your smoothie.

Nutrition: Calories: 395 Fat: 39g Carbohydrates: 11g Protein: 5.2g

4. __Morning Eggplant Soup__

Preparation time: 20 minutes

Cooking time: 15 minutes

Servings: 8

Ingredients:

- 1 large eggplant, washed and cubed
- 1 tomato, seeded and chopped
- 1 small onion, diced
- 2 tablespoons parsley, chopped
- 2 tablespoons extra virgin olive oil
- 2 tablespoons distilled white vinegar
- ½ cup cashew cheese
- Salt as needed

Directions:

1. Preheat your outdoor grill to medium-high. Pierce the eggplant a few times using a knife/fork. Cook the eggplants on your grill for about 15 minutes until they are charred.
2. Keep them on the side and allow them to cool. Remove the skin from the eggplant and dice the pulp.
3. Transfer the pulp to a mixing bowl and add parsley, onion, tomato, olive oil, feta cheese, and vinegar Mix well and chill for 1 hour.

4. Season with salt, and enjoy!

Nutrition: Calories: 99 Fat: 7g Carbohydrates: 7g
Protein:3.4g

5. <u>Roasted Garlic Soup</u>

Preparation time: 15 minutes

Cooking time: 60 minutes

Servings:10

Ingredients:

- 1 tablespoon olive oil
- 2 bulbs garlic, peeled
- 3 shallots, chopped
- 1 large head cauliflower, chopped
- 6 cups vegetable broth
- Salt and pepper to taste

Directions:

1. Preheat your oven to 400 degrees Fahrenheit. Slice ¼ inch top of the garlic bulb and place it in aluminum foil. Grease with olive oil and roast in the oven for 35 minutes.
2. Squeeze the flesh out of the roasted garlic. Heat oil in a saucepan and add shallots, Sauté for 6 minutes. Add garlic and remaining ingredients.
3. Cover the pan, then adjust the heat to low. Let it cook for 15-20 minutes.

4. Use an immersion blender to puree the mixture—season soup with salt and pepper. Serve and enjoy!

Nutrition: Calories: 142 Fat: 8g Carbohydrates: 3.4g Protein: 4g

6. Roasted Cashew and Almond Butter Delight

Preparation time: 5 minutes

Cooking time: 12 minutes

Servings: 1 & ½ cup

Ingredients:

- 1 cup almonds, blanched
- 1/3 cup cashew nuts
- 2 tablespoons coconut oil
- Salt as needed
- ½ teaspoon cinnamon

Directions:

1. Preheat your oven to 350 degrees Fahrenheit. Bake almonds and cashews for 12 minutes. Let them cool.
2. Move to a food processor and put the remaining fixings. Add oil and keep blending until smooth. Serve and enjoy!

Nutrition: Calories: 205 Fat: 19g Carbohydrates: g Protein: 2.8g

7. __Cashew Cheese and Walnut Crumbles__

Preparation time: 10 minutes

Cooking time: 8 minutes

Servings: 10

Ingredients:

- 6 ounces cashew cheese
- 2 tablespoons walnuts, chopped
- 1 tablespoon unsalted butter
- ½ tablespoon fresh thyme chopped

Directions:

1. Preheat your oven to 350 degrees Fahrenheit. Prepare your two large rimmed baking sheets, then line with parchment.
2. Add cheese, butter to a food processor and blend; add walnuts to the mix and pulse. Take a tablespoon and scoop mix onto a baking sheet.
3. Top with chopped thyme. Bake for 8 minutes, transfer to a cooling rack. Let it cool for 30 minutes. Serve and enjoy!

Nutrition: Calories: 80 Fat: 3g Carbohydrates: 7g Protein: 7g

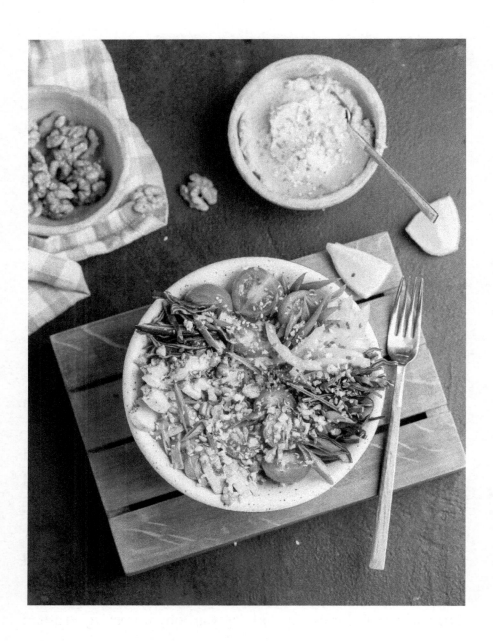

LUNCH

8. Thai Sweet Potato Noodles

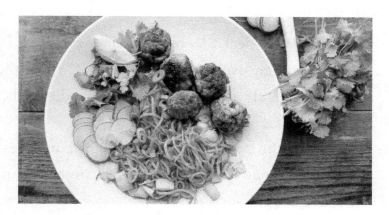

Preparation Time: 10 Minutes

Cooking Time: 24 Minutes

Servings: 4

Ingredients:

- 8 oz. Tofu, extra-firm
- 2 Sweet Potato, medium & spiralized
- 2 ½ tbsp. Sesame Oil, toasted
- 3 cups Baby Spinach
- ¼ cup Cashews, unsalted & chopped
- 1 cup Red Pepper, thinly sliced
- ½ cup Coconut Milk, light
- 3/4 tsp. Salt

- 3 tbsp. Almond Butter
- ½ cup Water
- 4 Lime Wedges
- 2 tbsp. Curry Paste

Directions:

1. To begin with, heat 1 ½ tablespoon of oil into a large-sized saucepan over medium-high heat. Once the oil becomes hot, stir in the sweet potato noodles, salt, and bell pepper.

2. Next, cook the sweet potato noodles for 4 minutes and then pour ¼ cup of water into them. Cover the pan and cook the noodles for 3 minutes.

3. After that, remove the lid and cook for a further 2 minutes. Now, add the spinach to the sweet potato mixture and cook until wilted.

4. Remove the mixture from the heat to a plate. Set it aside. Then, spoon in the remaining oil and fry the tofu in it while stirring it occasionally.

5. Next, mix coconut milk, curry paste, almond butter, salt, and remaining water in another bowl until combined well. Finally, pour ½ cup of the sauce into the sweet potato noodles mixture and toss well.

6. Distribute the noodles among the serving bowls and top it with the tofu, cashews, and remaining sauce. Serve along with lime wedges.

Nutrition: Calories: 357Proteins: 12g Carbohydrates: 27g Fat: 24.4g

9. Tahini Lemon Quinoa

Preparation Time: 10 Minutes

Cooking Time: 50 Minutes

Servings: 4

Ingredients:

- 1 cup Quinoa
- ¼ cup Lime Juice, fresh
- 15 oz. Chickpeas
- 1 cup Mint Leaves, packed & fresh
- Zest & Juice of 1 Lemon
- 1 tbsp. Agave Nectar
- 1 lb. Asparagus
- Salt & pepper, as needed
- ½ cup Tahini
- ¼ cup Pistachios, chopped

Directions:

1. First, mix chickpeas, pepper, lemon zest, salt, and lemon juice in a medium-sized mixing bowl and set it aside for 20 minutes. If possible, you can refrigerate overnight. Drain.
2. In the meantime, cook the quinoa by following the instructions given on the packet.

3. After that, place lime juice, ¼ teaspoon of salt, ½ cup of water, tahini, agave nectar, and mint in the high-speed blender. Blend for 1 minute or until you get a smooth dressing.

4. Next, with a peeler, make ribbons out of asparagus. Finally, combine quinoa along with shaved asparagus and chickpeas.

5. Garnish it with the pistachios and drizzle the dressing over it before serving.

Nutrition: Calories: 525 Proteins: 20g Carbohydrates: 64g

10. Tofu Bowl

Preparation Time: 10 Minutes

Cooking Time: 30 Minutes

Servings: 4

Ingredients:

- 1 Cucumber, seedless & chopped
- 14 oz. Tofu, extra-firm
- 3 tbsp. Cornstarch
- 1 cup Quinoa, cooked
- ½ of 1 Red Onion, small & sliced thinly
- 1 tbsp. Olive Oil
- ¼ cup Red Wine Vinegar
- Parsley leaves, fresh & chopped
- ¼ cup Thai Sweet Chili Sauce
- 2 tbsp. Cashews halved & roasted

Directions:

1. For making this delightful fare, you need to slice ¼ inch thick tofu pieces. After that, keep the tofu pieces between two chopping boards and then place heavy items on top of the boards for 10 minutes.
2. Next, place the onion in water for 8 to 10 minutes in such a way that they are soaked. Then, combine the

Thai sweet chili sauce, ¼ teaspoon of salt, and olive oil in a medium bowl with a whisker until mixed well.

3. Now, pat the onion with a paper towel and then place it along with cucumber and half of vinegar. Once combined, coat the tofu pieces with the cornstarch and set it aside.

4. Next, heat oil in a medium-sized skillet over medium-high heat, and once it becomes hot, stir in the tofu gently.

5. Fry the tofu for 3 minutes or until they are golden brown. Transfer the cooked pieces to a paper towel-lined plate.

6. Finally, divide the quinoa mixture between four serving bowls and top it with tofu, salad, parsley, and roasted cashews.

Nutrition: Calories: 440Proteins: 18g Carbohydrates: 45g Fat: 20g

11.   Linguine with Wild Mushrooms

Preparation Time: 10 Minutes

Cooking Time: 30 Minutes

Servings: 6

Ingredients:

- 2 Green Onions, sliced thinly
- 1 lb. Linguine
- ¼ cup Nutritional Yeast
- 6 tbsp. Oil
- 3 Garlic cloves, chopped finely
- 12 oz. Mixed Mushrooms, sliced thinly
- ½ tsp. Salt
- ¾ tsp. Black Pepper, grounded

Directions:

1. To start with, cook the linguine by following the instructions given on the packet.
2. Reserve ¾ cup of the pasta water while draining the pasta. Transfer the cooked pasta to a pot.
3. Then, heat oil in a large saucepan over medium-high heat. To this, stir in the mushrooms and garlic.
4. Sauté for 4 minutes or until the mushrooms are tender. Stir frequently. Next, transfer the mushrooms to the

linguine and the nutritional yeast, salt, pepper, and ¾ cup of the water.

5. Give a good stir until everything comes together. Finally, top it with green onions.

Nutrition: Calories: 430 Proteins: 15g Carbohydrates: 62g Fat: 15g

12. **<u>Ramen Noodle Salad</u>**

Preparation Time: 10 Minutes

Cooking Time: 15 Minutes

Servings: 4

Ingredients:

For the salad:

- 1 cup White Cabbage, shredded
- 1 Avocado, diced
- 4 Scallion, medium & sliced thinly
- 2 Carrot, medium & shredded
- ½ cup Peanuts, roasted & salted
- 1 cup Edamame, shelled & frozen
- 1 cup Red Cabbage, shredded
- 4 oz. Ramen Noodles
- 1 Mango, diced
- 1 cup Mung Bean Sprouts

For the dressing:

- 2 tbsp. Sesame Oil, toasted
- 2 tbsp. Maple Syrup
- Juice from 2 Limes
- 2 tbsp. Soy Sauce

Directions:

1. First, cook the noodles by following the instructions given by the manufacturer. Once cooked, wash them under cold water.

2. After that, make the dressing by mixing lime juice, sesame oil, soy sauce, and maple syrup in a small bowl until combined well.

3. Finally, toss all the salad ingredients to a large mixing bowl along with the noodles and dressing. Serve and enjoy.

Nutrition: Calories: 517Proteins: 18g Carbohydrates: 64g Fat: 26g

13. Asian Flavored Seitan

Preparation Time: 10 Minutes

Cooking Time: 20 Minutes

Servings: 6

Ingredients:

For the seitan:

- 1 ½ tbsp. Vegetable Oil
- 1 lb. Seitan, cubed into 1-inch pieces

For the sauce:

- 2 tsp. Vegetable Oil
- 2 tsp. Cornstarch
- ½ tsp. Garlic, grated
- 2 tbsp. Cold Water
- 1/3 tsp. Red Pepper Flakes
- ½ tsp. Ginger, grated
- ½ cup Coconut Sugar
- ½ cup Vegetable Broth
- ½ cup Soy Sauce

Directions:

1. For making this tasty Asian fare, you need to heat a medium-sized skillet over medium-high heat. To this, spoon in the oil and once it becomes hot, stir in the

garlic and ginger while stirring it continuously for half a minute.

2. Then, add red pepper flakes to it and sauté for another one minute or until aromatic. Next, pour the soy sauce and coconut sugar into the mixture. Mix well.

3. Now, lower the heat to medium-low and allow it to simmer for 7 minutes or until the sugar has completely dissolved.

4. Combine the cornstarch and water in another bowl until mixed well, and then pour this into the skillet. Combine.

5. Cook for another 3 minutes and lower the heat to low. Allow the mixture to simmer within 3 minutes or until the sauce is glossy and thickened. Tip: Keep simmering until the seitan gets added.

6. Heat the oil in a medium-sized saucepan over medium-high heat, and to this, add the seitan. Cook them for 5 minutes or until lightly browned.

7. Finally, add the seitan to the sauce and gently toss so that the seitan coats the sauce well. Garnish with sesame seeds and scallions.

Nutrition: Calories: 324 Proteins: 29g Carbohydrates: 33g Fat: 8g

14. **Vegan BLT**

Preparation Time: 10 Minutes

Cooking Time: 20 Minutes

Servings: 6

Ingredients:

- 3 ½ oz. Tempeh
- ¼ of 1 Avocado, mashed
- 1 ½ tbsp. Tamari
- 1 Tomato, sliced thinly
- 2 tsp. Liquid Smoke
- 1 tsp. Hot Sauce
- 2 slices of Sourdough Bread
- Few Salad leaves
- 2 tsp. Vegan Mayonnaise

Directions:

1. Begin by marinating the tempeh in tamari and liquid smoke. Set it aside for a few minutes. After that, heat the oil in a medium-sized saucepan over medium-high heat.

2. Once the oil becomes hot, stir in the tempeh and fry them for 2 to 3 minutes or golden-brown color and slightly crispy.

3. Next, spoon in the marinade over the tempeh and toss well. Then, toast the bread. Now, spread the combo of hot sauce and vegan mayonnaise on one side of the sourdough bread slice.

4. Spread your mashed avocado on the other slice. Finally, layer the bread with the tempeh, salad leaves, and tomato.

Nutrition: Calories: 503 Proteins: 30.9g Carbohydrates: 54g Fat: 21.1g

DINNER

15. **Curried Apple**

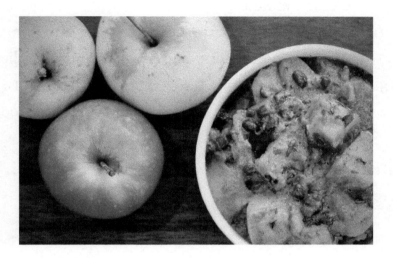

Preparation time: 15 minutes

Cooking time: 1 hour & 20 minutes

Servings: 4

Ingredients:

- 1 tablespoon fresh lemon juice
- ½ cup of water
- 2 apples, Fuji or Honeycrisp, cored and thinly sliced into rings
- 1 teaspoon curry powder

Directions:

1. Warm your oven to 200 Fahrenheit, take a rimmed baking sheet and line with parchment paper. Take a bowl and mix in lemon juice and water, add apples and soak for 2 minutes.
2. Pat them dry and arrange in a single layer on your baking sheet, dust curry powder on top of apple slices.
3. Bake within 45 minutes, after 45 minutes, turn the apples and bake for 45 minutes more. Let them cool for extra crispiness, serve and enjoy!

Nutrition: Calories: 240 Fat: 13g Carbohydrates: 20g Protein: 6g

16. <u>Cilantro and Avocado Platter</u>

Preparation time: 15 minutes

Cooking time: 0 minutes

Servings: 6

Ingredients:

- 2 avocados, peeled, pitted and diced
- 1 sweet onion, chopped
- 1 green bell pepper, chopped
- 1 large ripe tomato, chopped
- ¼ cup of fresh cilantro, chopped
- ½ a lime, juiced
- Salt and pepper as needed

Directions:

1. Take a medium-sized bowl and add onion, bell pepper, tomato, avocados, lime and cilantro. Mix well and give it a toss. Season with salt and pepper according to your taste. Serve and enjoy!

Nutrition: Calories: 126 Fat: 10g Carbohydrates: 10g Protein: 2g

17.   <u>Brussels' Fever</u>

Preparation time: 15 minutes

Cooking time: 20 minutes

Servings: 4

Ingredients:

- 2 tablespoons olive oil
- 1 yellow onion, chopped
- 2 pounds Brussels sprouts, trimmed and halved
- 4 cups vegetable stock
- ¼ cup coconut cream

Directions:

1. Take a pot and place it over medium heat. Add oil and let it heat up. Add onion and stir cook for 3 minutes. Add Brussels sprouts and stir, cook for 2 minutes.
2. Add stock and black pepper, stir and bring to a simmer. Cook for 20 minutes more. Make the soup creamy using an immersion blender.
3. Add coconut cream and stir well. Ladle into soup bowls and serve. Enjoy!

Nutrition: Calories: 200 Fat: 11g Carbohydrates: 6g Protein: 11g

18. Zucchini and Onions Platter

Preparation time: 15 minutes

Cooking time: 45 minutes

Servings: 4

Ingredients:

- 3 large zucchinis, julienned
- 1 cup cherry tomatoes, halved
- ½ cup basil
- 2 red onions, thinly sliced
- ¼ teaspoon sunflower seeds
- 1 teaspoon cayenne pepper
- 2 tablespoons lemon juice

Directions:

1. Create zucchini zoodles by using a vegetable peeler and shaving the zucchini with peeler lengthwise, until you get to the core and seeds.
2. Turn zucchini and repeat until you have long strips. Discard seeds. Lay strips on cutting board and slice lengthwise to your desired thickness.
3. Mix zoodles in a bowl with onion, basil and tomatoes, and toss. Sprinkle sunflower seeds and cayenne pepper on top.

4. Drizzle lemon juice. Serve and enjoy!

Nutrition: Calories: 156 Fat: 8g Carbohydrates: 6g Protein: 7g

19. Coconut and Cauliflower Rice with Chili

Preparation time: 15 minutes

Cooking time: 20 minutes

Servings: 4

Ingredients:

- 3 cups cauliflower, riced
- 2/3 cups full-fat coconut almond milk
- 1-2 teaspoons sriracha paste
- ¼- ½ teaspoon onion powder
- Sunflower seeds as needed
- Fresh basil for garnish

Directions:

1. Take a pan and place it over medium-low heat. Add all of the ingredients and stir them until fully combined. Cook for about 5-10 minutes, making sure that the lid is on.
2. Remove the lid and keep cooking until any excess liquid goes away. Once the rice is soft and creamy, enjoy it!

Nutrition: Calories: 95 Fat: 7g Carbohydrates: 4g Protein: 1g

20. Collard Greens 'N Tofu

Preparation time: 15 minutes

Cooking time: 10 minutes

Servings: 4

Ingredients:

- 2 pounds of collard greens, rinsed, chopped
- 1 cup water
- 1/2 pound of tofu, chopped
- Salt to taste
- Pepper powder to taste
- Crushed red chili to taste

Direction:

1. Place a large skillet over medium-high heat. Add oil. Put the tofu and cook until brown. Add rest of the fixings and mix well. Cook until greens wilts and almost dry.

Nutrition: Calories: 49 Carbs: 9g Fat: 1g Protein: 4g

21. **Cassoulet**

Preparation time: 15 minutes

Cooking time: 52 minutes

Servings: 4

Ingredients:

- ¼ cup olive oil, divided
- 4 ounces quit-the-cluck seitan, chopped
- 1/3 of a smoky vegan sausage, chopped
- 1½ cups chopped onion
- 2 ounces minced shiitake mushrooms
- 2 large carrots, peeled, sliced into ¼-inch (6 mm) rounds
- 2 stalks celery, chopped
- 1½ cups vegetable broth, divided
- 1 teaspoon liquid smoke
- 3 cans (each 15 ounces) white beans of choice, drained and rinsed
- 1 can (14.5 ounces) diced tomatoes, undrained
- 2 tablespoons tomato paste
- 1 tablespoon tamari
- 1 tablespoon no chicken bouillon paste, or 2 bouillon cubes, crumbled
- 2 tablespoons minced fresh parsley

- 2 teaspoons dried thyme
- ½ teaspoon dried rosemary salt and pepper
- 2 cups fresh bread crumbs
- ½ cup panko crumbs

Directions:

1. Preheat the oven to 375°f. Heat-up 1 tablespoon of olive oil in a large skillet over medium heat.
2. Add the seitan and vegan sausage. Cook for 4 to 6 minutes, occasionally stirring, until browned. Transfer to a plate and set aside.
3. Add the onion and a pinch of salt to the same skillet. Cook within 5 to 7 minutes until translucent. Transfer to the same plate.
4. Add the shiitakes, carrots, and celery to the skillet and cook for 2 minutes. Add 1 tablespoon vegetable broth and the liquid smoke. Cook for 2 to 3 minutes, stirring until the liquid is absorbed or evaporated.
5. Return the seitan and onions to the skillet and add the beans, tomatoes, tomato paste, tamari, bouillon, parsley, thyme, rosemary, and remaining broth.
6. Cook for 3 to 4 minutes, stirring to combine. Flavor with salt and pepper to taste and transfer to a large casserole pan.

7. Toss together the fresh bread crumbs, panko crumbs, and the remaining 3 tablespoons olive oil in a small bowl. Spread evenly over the bean mixture.
8. Bake within 30 to 35 minutes until the crumbs are browned.

Nutrition: Calories: 636 Carbs: 68g Fat: 30g Protein: 21g

22. **Mean Bean Minestrone**

Preparation time: 15 minutes

Cooking time: 36 minutes

Servings: 6

Ingredients:

- 1 tablespoon olive oil
- 1/3 cup chopped red onion
- 4 cloves garlic, grated or pressed
- 1 leek, white & light green parts, trimmed and chopped (about 4 ounces)
- 2 carrots, peeled and minced (about 4 ounces)
- 2 ribs of celery, minced (about 2 ounces)
- 2 yellow squashes, trimmed and chopped (about 8 ounces)
- 1 green bell pepper, trimmed and chopped (about 8 ounces)
- 1 tablespoon tomato paste
- 1 teaspoon dried oregano
- 1 teaspoon dried basil
- 1/3 teaspoon smoked paprika
- ¼ teaspoon cayenne pepper, or to taste
- 2 cans (each 15 ounces) diced fire-roasted tomatoes
- 4 cups vegetable broth, more if needed

- 3 cups cannellini beans, or other white beans
- 2 cups cooked farro, or other whole grain or pasta
- Salt, to taste
- Nut and seed sprinkles, for garnish, optional and to taste

Directions:

1. In a large pot, add the oil, onion, garlic, leek, carrots, celery, yellow squash, bell pepper, tomato paste, oregano, basil, paprika, and cayenne pepper.
2. Cook it on medium-high heat, stirring often until the vegetables start to get tender, about 6 minutes. Add the tomatoes and broth. Bring to a boil, lower the heat, cover with a lid, and simmer 15 minutes.
3. Add the beans and simmer another 10 minutes. Add the farro and simmer 5 more minutes to heat the farro.
4. Put extra broth if you prefer a thinner soup and adjust seasoning if needed. Add nut and seed sprinkles on each portion upon serving, if desired.

Nutrition: Calories: 130 Carbs: 24g Fat: 2g Protein: 4g

SNACKS

23. Loaded Guacamole

Preparation time: 15 minutes

Cooking time: 0 minutes

Servings: 2

Ingredients:

- 1 avocado, halved and pitted
- 1 tomato, diced small
- 1 scallion, white & light green parts only, sliced
- 1 garlic clove, minced
- 2 tablespoons freshly squeezed lime juice
- Pinch salt
- Pinch freshly ground black pepper
- Pinch red pepper flakes (optional)
- Tortilla chips (optional, for serving)

Directions:

1. Spoon the avocado flesh into your medium bowl, and mash it with a fork. Stir in the tomato, scallion, garlic, lime juice, salt, pepper, and red pepper flakes (if using). Enjoy this with tortilla chips, if you like.

Nutrition: Calories: 74Protein: 1gFat: 6gCarbohydrates: 7g

24. Sliding-Scale Nachos

Preparation time: 15 minutes

Cooking time: 5-10 minutes

Servings: 1

Ingredients:

- 1 (2-ounce) bag tortilla chips
- ½ cup canned black beans, drained and rinsed
- 1 teaspoon olive oil
- 1 teaspoon chili powder
- Salt
- 1 tomato, diced
- 1 scallion, sliced, white & light green parts
- ½ bell pepper, any color, diced
- Sliced jalapeño pepper (optional)
- ¼ cup grated vegan cheese (optional)
- Optional toppings: Loaded Guacamole, Sour Cream, salsa, and/or cheese sauce

Directions:

1. Warm your oven or toaster oven to 350°F. Lay the tortilla chips on a rimmed baking sheet or toaster oven tray.

2. In a small bowl, stir together the black beans, olive oil, chili powder, and a pinch of salt. Sprinkle the beans over the chips.

3. Top with the tomato, scallion, bell pepper, jalapeño (if using), and cheese (if using). Bake within 5 to 10 minutes, until the chips are slightly browned around the edges and the cheese melts. Enjoy your nachos with any extra toppings you like.

Nutrition: Calories: 538Protein:14gFat: 22gCarbohydrates: 72g

25. <u>Homemade Fries</u>

Preparation time: 15 minutes

Cooking time: 20-30 minutes

Servings: 2

Ingredients:

- 4 cups peeled root vegetable matchsticks
- 1 tablespoon olive oil
- Salt

Directions:

1. Warm your oven or toaster oven to 350°F. On a rimmed baking sheet or toaster oven tray, toss the vegetables with the olive oil and salt, then spread them out in a single layer.
2. Bake for 20 to 30 minutes, turning occasionally, until tender and browned.

Nutrition: Calories: 331Protein: 6gFat: 7gCarbohydrates: 63g

26. <u>Barbecue Cauliflower Wings</u>

Preparation time: 15 minutes

Cooking time: 40 minutes

Servings: 4

Ingredients:

- Olive oil, for preparing the baking sheet (optional)
- ½ cup all-purpose flour
- 2 teaspoons garlic powder
- Salt
- Freshly ground black pepper
- ½ cup nondairy milk
- ¼ cup water
- 2 cups small cauliflower florets
- ½ cup Simple Barbecue Sauce
- ½ cup Creamy Tahini Dressing or Caesar Dressing

Directions:

1. Warm your oven or toaster oven to 350°F. Coat a rimmed baking sheet with olive oil or line it with parchment paper or a silicone mat.
2. In a large bowl, combine the flour and garlic powder, and season to taste with salt and pepper. Whisk in the milk and water until thoroughly combined.

3. Dunk the cauliflower chunks into the batter, making sure they're fully coated, then place them on the prepared baking sheet in a single layer. Bake for 20 minutes.
4. Drizzle the cauliflower with barbecue sauce, and carefully turn to coat. Bake for 20 minutes more.
5. Remove the cauliflower from the oven, and let it cool for a few minutes. Serve with your choice of dressing for dipping.

Nutrition: Calories: 274Protein: 9gFat: 11gCarbohydrates: 39g

27. **Corn Fritters**

Preparation time: 15 minutes

Cooking time: 10 minutes

Servings: 2

Ingredients:

- ¾ cup corn kernels, thawed if frozen, drained if canned
- 1 scallion, white & light green parts only, sliced
- ¼ cup all-purpose flour
- ¼ teaspoon salt
- 2 tablespoons nondairy milk
- 1 tablespoon olive oil, + more as needed

Directions:

1. Stir the corn, scallion, flour, and salt in a large bowl. Stir in the milk. The mixture should be pretty thick and just barely sticking together. Form it into two loose patties.

2. Heat the olive oil in a large skillet over medium heat. Put the fritters, and cook for 2 to 3 minutes until browned. Flip and cook for 2 to 3 minutes more, adding more oil as needed. Don't cook too long or the corn might pop!

Nutrition: Calories: 203Protein: 5gFat: 8gCarbohydrates: 31g

VEGETABLES

28. Glazed Curried Carrots

Preparation Time: 5 minutes

Cooking Time: 15 minutes

Serving: 6

Ingredient:

- 1-pound carrots
- 2 tablespoons olive oil
- 2 tablespoons curry powder
- 2 tablespoons pure maple syrup
- Juice of ½ lemon

Direction

1. Cook carrots with water over medium-high heat for 10 minutes. Drain and return them to the pan over medium-low heat.
2. Stir in the olive oil, curry powder, maple syrup, and lemon juice.

3. Cook, stirring constantly, until the liquid reduces, about 5 minutes. Season well and serve immediately.

Nutrition: 91 Calories 5g Fiber 9g Protein

29. **Pepper Medley**

Preparation Time: 10 minutes

Cooking Time: 15 minutes

Serving: 4

Ingredient:

- 3 tablespoons olive oil
- 1 red bell pepper, sliced
- 1 orange bell pepper, sliced
- 1 yellow bell pepper, sliced
- 1 green bell pepper, sliced
- 2 garlic cloves, minced
- 3 tablespoons red wine vinegar
- 2 tablespoons chopped fresh basil

Direction:

1. Warm up olive oil over medium-high heat. Stir in the bell peppers and cook, stir, for 7 to 10 minutes. Cook garlic for 30 seconds. Add the vinegar, using a spoon to scrape any browned bits off the bottom of the pan.
2. Simmer until the vinegar reduces, 2 to 3 minutes. Season. Stir in the basil and serve immediately.

Nutrition: 96 Calories 3g Fiber 5g Protein

SALAD

30. <u>Spinach and Mashed Tofu Salad</u>

Preparation Time: 20 minutes

Cooking Time: 0 minutes

Servings: 4

Ingredients:

- 2 8-oz. blocks firm tofu, drained
- 4 cups baby spinach leaves
- 4 tbsp. cashew butter
- 1½ tbsp. soy sauce
- 1tbsp ginger, chopped
- 1 tsp. red miso paste
- 2 tbsp. sesame seeds
- 1 tsp. organic orange zest
- 1 tsp. nori flakes
- 2 tbsp. water

Directions:

1. Use paper towels to absorb any excess water left in the tofu before crumbling both blocks into small pieces.

2. In a large bowl, combine the mashed tofu with the spinach leaves.

3. Mix the remaining ingredients in another small bowl and, if desired, add the optional water for a smoother dressing.

4. Pour this dressing over the mashed tofu and spinach leaves.

5. Transfer the bowl to the fridge and allow the salad to chill for up to one hour. Doing so will guarantee a better flavor. Or, the salad can be served right away. Enjoy!

Nutrition: Calories 623Total Fat 30.5gSaturated Fat 5.8g Cholesterol 0mgSodium 2810mgTotal Carbohydrate 48gDietary Fiber 5.9gTotal Sugars 3gProtein 48.4gVitamin D 0mcgCalcium 797mgIron 22mgPotassium 2007mg

GRAINS

31. Peppery Black Beans

Preparation Time: 10 minutes

Cooking Time: 33 to 34 minutes

Servings: 4

Ingredients:

- 1 red bell pepper, deseeded and chopped
- 1 medium yellow onion, peeled and chopped
- 2 jalapeño peppers, deseeded and minced
- 4 cloves garlic, peeled and minced
- 1 tablespoon thyme
- 1 tablespoon curry powder
- 1½ teaspoons ground allspice
- 1 teaspoon freshly ground black pepper
- 1 (15-ounce / 425-g) can diced tomatoes
- 4 cups cooked black beans

Directions:

1. Add the red bell pepper and onion to a saucepan and sauté over medium heat for 10 minutes, or until the onion is softened. Add water 1 to 2

tablespoons at a time to keep the vegetables from sticking to the pan.

2. Stir in the jalapeño peppers, garlic, thyme, curry powder, allspice and black pepper. Cook for 3 to 4 minutes, then add the tomatoes and black beans. Cook over medium heat for 20 minutes, covered.

3. Serve immediately.

Nutrition: calories: 283fat: 1.7gcarbs: 52.8gprotein: 17.4gfiber: 19.8g

32.   Walnut, Coconut, and Oat Granola

Preparation Time: 15 minutes

Cooking Time: 1 hour 40 minutes

Servings: 4

Ingredients:

- 1 cup chopped walnuts
- 1 cup unsweetened, shredded coconut
- 2 cups rolled oats
- 1 teaspoon ground cinnamon
- 2 tablespoons hemp seeds
- 2 tablespoons ground flaxseeds
- 2 tablespoons chia seeds
- ¾ teaspoon salt (optional)
- ¼ cup maple syrup
- ¼ cup water
- 1 teaspoon vanilla extract
- ½ cup dried cranberries

Directions:

1. Preheat the oven to 250°F (120°C). Line a baking sheet with parchment paper.
2. Mix the walnuts, coconut, rolled oats, cinnamon, hemp seeds, flaxseeds, chia seeds, and salt (if desired) in a bowl.

3. Combine the maple syrup and water in a saucepan. Bring to a boil over medium heat, then pour in the bowl of walnut mixture.

4. Add the vanilla extract to the bowl of mixture. Stir to mix well. Pour the mixture in the baking sheet, then level with a spatula so the mixture coats the bottom evenly.

5. Place the baking sheet in the preheated oven and bake for 90 minutes or until browned and crispy. Stir the mixture every 15 minutes.

6. Remove the baking sheet from the oven. Allow to cool for 10 minutes, then serve with dried cranberries on top.

Nutrition: calories: 1870 fat: 115.8gcarbs: 238.0gprotein: 59.8gfiber: 68.9g

LEGUMES

33. Traditional Indian Rajma Dal

Preparation Time: 10 minutes

Cooking Time: 10 minutes

Servings: 4

Ingredients:

- 3 tablespoons sesame oil
- 1 teaspoon ginger, minced
- 1 teaspoon cumin seeds
- 1 teaspoon coriander seeds
- 1 large onion, chopped
- 1 celery stalk, chopped
- 1 teaspoon garlic, minced
- 1 cup tomato sauce
- 1 teaspoon garam masala
- 1/2 teaspoon curry powder
- 1 small cinnamon stick
- 1 green chili, seeded and minced
- 2 cups canned red kidney beans, drained
- 2 cups vegetable broth
- Kosher salt and ground black pepper, to taste

Directions

1. In a saucepan, heat the sesame oil over medium-high heat; now, sauté the ginger, cumin seeds and coriander seeds until fragrant or about 30 seconds or so.
2. Add in the onion and celery and continue to sauté for 3 minutes more until they've softened.
3. Add in the garlic and continue to sauté for 1 minute longer.
4. Stir the remaining ingredients into the saucepan and turn the heat to a simmer. Continue to cook for 10 to 12 minutes or until thoroughly cooked. Serve warm and enjoy!

Nutrition: Per serving: Calories: 443; Fat: 19.2g; Carbs: 52.2g; Protein: 18.1g

34. **Red Kidney Bean Salad**

Preparation Time: 10 minutes

Cooking Time: 10 minutes

Servings: 4

Ingredients:

- 3/4-pound red kidney beans, soaked overnight
- 2 bell peppers, chopped
- 1 carrot, trimmed and grated
- 3 ounces frozen or canned corn kernels, drained
- 3 heaping tablespoons scallions, chopped
- 2 cloves garlic, minced
- 1 red chile pepper, sliced
- 1/2 cup extra-virgin olive oil
- 2 tablespoons apple cider vinegar
- 2 tablespoons fresh lemon juice
- Sea salt and ground black pepper, to taste
- 2 tablespoons fresh cilantro, chopped
- 2 tablespoons fresh parsley, chopped
- 2 tablespoons fresh basil, chopped

Directions

1. Cover the soaked beans with a fresh change of cold water and bring to a boil. Let it boil for about 10

minutes. Turn the heat to a simmer and continue to cook for 50 to 55 minutes or until tender.

2. Allow your beans to cool completely, then, transfer them to a salad bowl.

3. Add in the remaining ingredients and toss to combine well. Bon appétit!

Nutrition: Calories: 443; Fat: 19.2g; Carbs: 52.2g; Protein: 18.1g

BREAD & PIZZA

35. Keto Burger Buns

Preparation time: 10 minutes

Cooking time: 12 minutes

Servings: 6

Ingredients:

- 1 cup Almond Flour
- 1/4 cup Psyllium Husk Powder
- 1 teaspoon Baking Powder
- 1 cup Mozzarella Cheese
- 1/4 cup Cream Cheese
- 1 Egg
- tablespoon Sesame Seeds

Directions:

1. Preheat oven to 400-degree F.
2. Melt the two cheeses together in the microwave.
3. Blend the melted cheese together then stir in the egg.
4. Whisk together the almond flour, psyllium husk, and baking powder in a separate bowl.
5. Mix the dry ingredients into the cheese mixture until a dough is formed.

6. Divide the dough into 6 and roll each portion into a ball.
7. Top each ball with sesame seeds.
8. Arrange on a baking sheet lined with parchment and bake for 12 minutes.
9. Leave to cool for 10-15 minutes before slicing into halves.

Nutrition: Calories 216 Carbohydrates 5 g Fats 18 g Protein 10 g

36. Keto Pizza Crust

Preparation time: 10 minutes

Cooking time: 6 minutes

Servings: 8

Ingredients:

- 1 cup Almond Flour
- 2 cups Shredded Mozzarella
- 2 tablespoon Cream Cheese
- Pinch of Salt

Directions:

1. Combine both cheeses in a bowl and melt in the microwave.
2. Stir then gradually knead in the salt and almond flour.
3. Roll out to flatten in between sheets of parchment.
4. Bake at 350-degree F for 6 minutes.
5. Put choice of toppings on and bake for another 5-10 minutes.

Nutrition: Calories 165 Carbohydrates 3 g Fats 13 g Protein 9 g

SOUP AND STEW

37. Avocado Cucumber Soup

Preparation Time: 20 minutes

Cooking Time: 0 minutes

Servings: 3

Ingredients:

- 1 large cucumber, peeled and sliced
- ¾ cup water
- ¼ cup lemon juice
- 2 garlic cloves
- 6 green onion
- 2 avocados, pitted
- ½ tsp black pepper
- ½ tsp pink salt

Directions:

1. Add all ingredients into the blender and blend until smooth and creamy.
2. Place in refrigerator for 30 minutes.
3. Stir well and serve chilled.

Nutrition: Calories: 127 kcalFat: 6.6g Carbs: 13g Protein: 0.7g

38. <u>Garden Vegetable Stew</u>

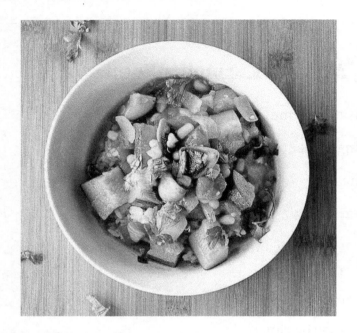

Preparation Time: 5 minutes

Cooking Time: 60 minutes

Servings: 4

Ingredients:

- 2 tablespoons olive oil
- 1 medium red onion, chopped
- 1 medium carrot, cut into 1/4-inch slices
- 1/2 cup dry white wine
- 3 medium new potatoes, unpeeled and cut into 1-inch pieces
- 1 medium red bell pepper, cut into 1/2-inch dice

- 11/2 cups vegetable broth
- 1 tablespoon minced fresh savory or 1 teaspoon dried

Directions:

1. In a large saucepan, heat the oil over medium heat. Add the onion and carrot, cover, and cook until softened, 7 minutes. Add the wine and cook, uncovered, for 5 minutes. Stir in the potatoes, bell pepper, and broth and bring to a boil. Reduce the heat to medium and simmer for 15 minutes.

2. Add the zucchini, yellow squash, and tomatoes. Season with salt and black pepper to taste, cover, and simmer until the vegetables are tender, 20 to 30 minutes. Stir in the corn, peas, basil, parsley, and savory. Taste, adjusting seasonings if necessary. Simmer to blend flavors, about 10 minutes more. Serve immediately.

Nutrition: Calories: 219 kcal Fat: 4.5g Carbs: 38.2g Protein: 6.4g

SAUCES, DRESSINGS & DIP

39. Spicy Avocado Mayonnaise

Preparation time: 10 minutes

Cooking time: 10 minutes

Servings: 8

Ingredients:

- 2 ripe avocados, pitted and peeled
- 1/4 jalapeno pepper, minced
- 2 tablespoon lemon juice
- 1/2 teaspoon onion powder
- 2 tablespoons fresh cilantro, chopped
- Salt to taste

Directions:

1. Add all **Ingredients:** to a food processor and blender until a smooth creamy consistency is achieved.

2. The jalapeno peppers can be foregone if you prefer a cooler mayo.

3. Can be enjoyed in sandwiches, on toast, as a topping, in veggie wraps and salads

Nutrition: Total fat: 9.8g Cholesterol: 0mg Sodium: 23mg

Total carbohydrates: 4.6g Dietary fiber: 3.4g Protein: 1g

40. Green Coconut Butter

Preparation time: 10 minutes

Cooking time: 10 minutes

Servings: 8

Ingredients:

- 2 cups unsweetened shredded coconut
- 2 teaspoon matcha powder
- 1 tablespoon coconut oil

Directions:

1. Add shredded coconut to a food processor and blend for 5 minutes or until a smooth but runny consistency is achieved.

2. Add matcha powder and olive oil. Blend for 1 more minute.

3. Can be stored in an airtight container at room temperature for up to 2 weeks. Makes a delicious fruit dip and can be added to smoothies, on pancakes and toast.

Nutrition: Total fat: 5.2g Cholesterol: 0mg Sodium: 3mg Total carbohydrates: 1.7g Dietary fiber: 1.2g Protein: 0.7g

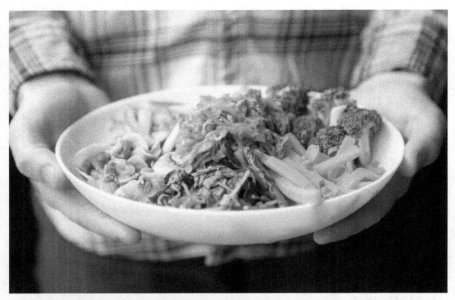

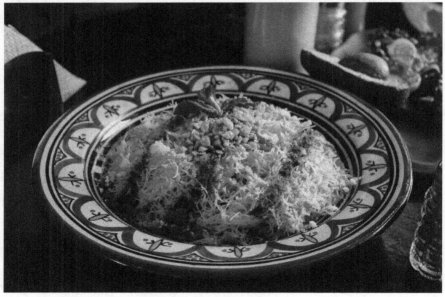

APPETIZER

41. <u>Curry White Bean Cup</u>

Preparation Time: 15 minutes

Cooking Time: 0 minutes

Servings: 4 servings

Ingredients:

- 1 can white beans
- 1 garlic clove
- 1 tablespoon lemon juice
- ¼ cup avocado oil
- 3 teaspoons curry powder
- ½ teaspoon paprika
- sea salt and black pepper to preference

Directions:

1. Add all fixings to a food processor and blend until smooth. Transfer to an airtight container and store in the refrigerator until ready to be consumed.

Nutrition: Calories 280Fat 14 g Protein 12 g Carbs 32 g

42. <u>**Vegan Onion Rings**</u>

Preparation Time: 30 minutes

Cooking Time: 10 minutes

Servings: 4 servings

Ingredients:

- 2 sweet onions, peeled
- 2/3 cup all-purpose flour
- 2/3 cup almond milk, unsweetened
- 1 teaspoon garlic powder
- 1 teaspoon smoked paprika powder
- 1 tablespoon nutritional yeast
- 1 cup panko breadcrumbs
- ¼ teaspoon salt

Directions:

2. Preheat oven to 350°F. Line a baking sheet with parchment paper. Combine flour, spices, nutritional yeast, and almond milk in a bowl. Stir well.
3. Place the breadcrumbs into a separate bowl. Cut the onions into ¼ inch rings and separate.
4. Coat each onion ring in the spices, then follow by dipping in the breadcrumbs. Lay the onion rings onto the baking sheet when finished.

5. Bake for 20 minutes. Remove the pan and flip each onion ring. Bake for an additional 10 minutes. Serve warm with additional dipping sauce if desired.

Nutrition: Calories 200Fat 1 g Protein 6 g Carbs 40 g

SMOOTHIES AND JUICES

43. Overnight Oats on the Go

Preparation Time: 5 minutes

Cooking Time: 5 minutes or Overnight

Servings: 1 serving

Ingredients:

Basic Overnight Oats

- ½ cup rolled oats, or quinoa flakes for gluten-free
- 1 tablespoon ground flaxseed, or chia seeds, or hemp hearts
- 1 tablespoon maple syrup, or coconut sugar (optional)
- ¼ teaspoon ground cinnamon (optional)

Topping Options

- 1 apple, chopped, and 1 tablespoon walnuts
- 2 tablespoons dried cranberries and 1 tablespoon pumpkin seeds
- 1 pear, chopped, and 1 tablespoon cashews
- 1 cup sliced grapes and 1 tablespoon sunflower seeds
- 1 banana, sliced, and 1 tablespoon peanut butter
- 2 tablespoons raisins and 1 tablespoon hazelnuts

- 1 cup berries and 1 tablespoon unsweetened coconut flakes

Directions:

1. Mix the oats, flax, maple syrup, and cinnamon (if using) in a bowl or to-go container (a travel mug or short thermos works beautifully).
2. Pour enough cool water over the oats to submerge them, and stir to combine. Leave to soak for a minimum of half an hour, or overnight.
3. Add your choice of toppings.

Nutrition: Calories: 244Total fat: 6gCarbs: 30gFiber: 6gProtein: 7g

44. **Zobo Drink**

Preparation Time: 5 minutes

Cooking Time: 10 minutes

Servings: 8

Ingredients:

- 2 cups dried hibiscus petals (zobo leaves), rinsed
- Pineapple rind from 1 pineapple
- 1 cup of granulated sugar
- 1 tsp. fresh ginger, grated
- 10 cups of water

Directions:

1. Add water, ginger, and sugar into the pot and mix well.
2. Then add zobo leaves and pineapple rind.
3. Cover and cook on High for 10 minutes. Open and discard solids.
4. Chill and serve.

Nutrition: Calories 65; Carbs 7g; Fat 2.6g; Protein 1.14g

DESSERTS

45. <u>Chocolate N'ice Cream</u>

Preparation time: 15 minutes

Cooking time: 0 minutes

Servings: 1

Ingredients:

- 2 frozen bananas, peeled and sliced
- 2 tablespoons coconut milk
- 1 teaspoon carob powder
- 1 teaspoon cocoa powder
- A pinch of grated nutmeg
- 1/8 teaspoon ground cardamom
- 1/8 teaspoon ground cinnamon
- 1 tablespoon chocolate curls

Directions:

1. Place all the fixings in the bowl of your food processor or high-speed blender. Blitz the ingredients until creamy or until your desired consistency is achieved.
2. Serve immediately or store in your freezer. Bon appétit!

Nutrition: Calories: 349Fat: 2.8Carbs: 84.1gProtein: 4.8g

46. <u>Raw Raspberry Cheesecake</u>

Preparation time: 3 hours & 15 minutes

Cooking time: 0 minutes

Servings: 9

Ingredients:

Crust:

- 2 cups almonds
- 1 cup fresh dates, pitted
- 1/4 teaspoon ground cinnamon

Filling:

- 2 cups raw cashews, soaked overnight & drained
- 14 ounces blackberries, frozen
- 1 tablespoon fresh lime juice
- 1/4 teaspoon crystallized ginger
- 1 can coconut cream
- 8 fresh dates, pitted

Directions:

1. In your food processor, blend the crust ingredients until the mixture comes together; press the crust into a lightly oiled springform pan.
2. Then, blend the filling layer until completely smooth. Spoon the filling onto the crust, creating a flat surface with a spatula.

3. Transfer the cake to your freezer for about 3 hours. Store in your freezer. Garnish with organic citrus peel. Bon appétit!

Nutrition: Calories: 385Fat: 22.9Carbs: 41.1gProtein: 10.8g

47. **Mini Lemon Tarts**

Preparation time: 15 minutes

Cooking time: 0 minutes

Servings: 9

Ingredients:

- 1 cup cashews
- 1 cup dates, pitted
- 1/2 cup coconut flakes
- 1/2 teaspoon anise, ground
- 3 lemons, freshly squeezed
- 1 cup coconut cream
- 2 tablespoons agave syrup

Directions:

1. Brush a muffin tin with a nonstick cooking oil. Blend the cashews, dates, coconut and anise in your food processor or a high-speed blender. Press the crust into the peppered muffin tin.
2. Then, blend the lemon, coconut cream and agave syrup. Spoon the cream into the muffin tin. Store in your freezer. Bon appétit!

Nutrition: Calories: 257Fat: 16.5Carbs: 25.4gProtein: 4g

48. Fluffy Coconut Blondies with Raisins

Preparation time: 15 minutes

Cooking time: 25 minutes

Servings: 9

Ingredients:

- 1 cup coconut flour
- 1 cup all-purpose flour
- 1/2 teaspoon baking powder
- 1/4 teaspoon salt
- 1 cup desiccated coconut, unsweetened
- 3/4 cup vegan butter, softened
- 1 ½ cups brown sugar
- 3 tablespoons applesauce
- 1/2 teaspoon vanilla extract
- 1/2 teaspoon ground anise
- 1 cup raisins, soaked for 15 minutes

Directions:

1. Warm your oven to 350 degrees F. Brush a baking pan with a nonstick cooking oil.
2. Thoroughly combine the flour, baking powder, salt and coconut. In another bowl, mix the butter, sugar, applesauce, vanilla and anise. Stir the butter mixture into the dry ingredients; stir to combine well.

3. Fold in the raisins. Press your batter into the baking pan. Bake within 25 minutes or until it is set in the middle. Place the cake on a wire rack to cool slightly. Bon appétit!

Nutrition: Calories: 365Fat: 18.5Carbs: 49gProtein: 2.1g

49. <u>Easy Chocolate Squares</u>

Preparation time: 1 hours & 15 minutes

Cooking time: 0 minutes

Servings: 20

Ingredients:

- 1 cup cashew butter
- 1 cup almond butter
- 1/4 cup coconut oil, melted
- 1/4 cup raw cacao powder
- 2 ounces dark chocolate
- 4 tablespoons agave syrup
- 1 teaspoon vanilla paste
- 1/4 teaspoon ground cinnamon
- 1/4 teaspoon ground cloves

Directions:

1. Process all the ingredients in your blender until uniform and smooth. Scrape the batter into a parchment-lined baking sheet.
2. Place it in your freezer for at least 1 hour to set. Cut into squares and serve. Bon appétit!

Nutrition: Calories: 187Fat: 13.8gCarbs: 15.1gProtein: 2.9g

50. <u>Strawberry Cheesecake Fat Bombs</u>

Preparation time: 4 hours & 15 minutes

Cooking time: 12 minutes

Servings: 12

Ingredients:

- Nonstick cooking spray
- 1/3 cup frozen strawberries
- 4½ tablespoons cream cheese
- 4½ tablespoons grass-fed butter
- 2 tablespoons powdered erythritol
- ½ teaspoon vanilla extract

Directions:

1. Spray the cups of a 12-cup mini muffin tin with cooking spray. In a small saucepan over low heat, bring the strawberries to a simmer and cook for 10 minutes while stirring, until all the excess liquid has evaporated, leaving just the strawberries. Set aside.
2. In the bowl of a stand mixer, combine the cream cheese, butter, erythritol, and vanilla, and mix on low for 3 to 4 minutes or until fluffy.
3. Pour in the strawberries and mix for another 1 to 2 minutes. Using a 2-inch cookie scoop, scoop the

mixture into the mini muffin cups. Place the muffin tin in the freezer to set for 4 hours.

4. Use a butter knife to remove the bombs from the tin (they should just pop right out) and place the bombs in a resealable freezer bag. Store in the freezer.

Nutrition: Calories: 58 Fat: 6g Protein: 0g

Carbs: 1g

Lightning Source UK Ltd.
Milton Keynes UK
UKHW050933060421
381487UK00016B/184